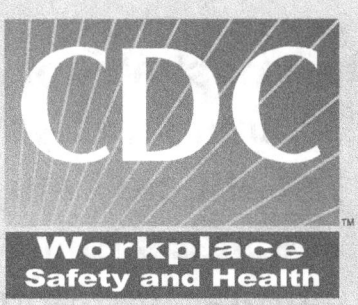

Evaluation of Cancer, Indoor Environmental Quality, and Potential Chemical Hazards at a Police Department

Kenneth W. Fent, PhD
Anthony Almazan, MD

Health Hazard Evaluation Report
HETA 2008-0237-3097
Cincinnati Police Department
Criminal Investigation Section
Cincinnati, Ohio
December 2009

Department of Health and Human Services
Centers for Disease Control and Prevention

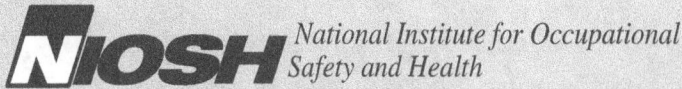

National Institute for Occupational
Safety and Health

CONTENTS

ABBREVIATIONS

ACGIH®	American Conference of Governmental Industrial Hygienists
AHU	Air handling unit
ANSI	American National Standards Institute
ASHRAE	American Society of Heating, Refrigerating, and Air-Conditioning Engineers
cc/min	Cubic centimeters per minute
CFR	Code of Federal Regulations
CIS	Criminal Investigation Section
CO_2	Carbon dioxide
CPD	Cincinnati Police Department
ft^3/min	Cubic feet per minute
ft/min	Feet per minute
ft^2	Square feet
HHE	Health hazard evaluation
HVAC	Heating, ventilating, and air-conditioning
IARC	International Agency for Research on Cancer
IEQ	Indoor environmental quality
LEV	Local exhaust ventilation
MDC	Minimum detectable concentration
mg/m^3	Milligrams per cubic meter
MQC	Minimum quantifiable concentration
NAICS	North American Industry Classification System
ND	Non-detectable
NIOSH	National Institute for Occupational Safety and Health
OEL	Occupational exposure limit
OSHA	Occupational Safety and Health Administration
PAH	Polycyclic aromatic hydrocarbon
PBZ	Personal breathing zone
PEL	Permissible exposure limit
PPE	Personal protective equipment
ppm	Parts per million
REL	Recommended exposure limit
RH	Relative humidity
STEL	Short term exposure limit
TLV®	Threshold limit value
TWA	Time-weighted average
WEEL	Workplace environmental exposure limit

The National Institute for Occupational Safety and Health (NIOSH) received a management request for a health hazard evaluation (HHE) at the Cincinnati Police Department (CPD), Criminal Investigation Section (CIS) in Cincinnati, Ohio. The HHE request was submitted because of concerns about cancer among current and former employees. NIOSH investigators evaluated the facility in November 2008.

What NIOSH Did

- We reviewed medical and work history information on CIS employees reported to have cancer.

- We interviewed employees about their symptoms or health concerns related to their work.

- We evaluated the heating, ventilating, and air conditioning (HVAC) and local exhaust ventilation (LEV) systems at the CPD.

- We checked to see if enough outdoor air was delivered to the occupied areas of the building.

- We sampled for chemicals used to process criminal evidence.

What NIOSH Found

- Cancers reported in current and former CIS employees were not likely related to workplace exposures.

- Eight of 13 employees we talked to had respiratory, neurological, or mucous membrane symptoms they believed were work related.

- All sampling results were below applicable occupational exposure limits.

- Several air filters in the HVAC and LEV systems needed to be replaced.

- The office areas did not receive enough outdoor air in the afternoon.

- Because of poor ventilation controls, chemical contaminants and nuisance odors could spread to other areas of the building.

- Criminalists were exposed to ethyl cyanoacrylate, a chemical in super glue, because of poor ventilation design and maintenance of the fuming chambers.

What Managers Can Do

- Encourage employees to learn more about cancer. Issues such as personal risk factors, screening programs, and steps to take to reduce their cancer risk should be stressed.

- Replace air filters in the HVAC and LEV systems routinely. These filters should be the proper size and meet manufacturer specifications.

- Increase the amount of outdoor air to occupied areas of the building while maintaining thermal comfort for the occupants.

- Add exhaust ventilation or maintain negative pressure in rooms that house chemicals or emit nuisance odors.

- Replace the super glue fuming chambers with units that minimize airborne ethyl cyanoacrylate exposures.

- Write a forensic laboratory health and safety plan. This plan should describe workplace hazards and list standard operating procedures, engineering controls, and personal protective equipment for each method used to process evidence.

- Organize a health and safety committee. This committee should consist of employee and management representatives who meet regularly to address health and safety concerns. This committee should also update the laboratory health and safety plan as needed.

What Employees Can Do

- Talk with your healthcare provider about your risk factors for cancer.

- Find out how you can decrease your risk of preventable cancers.

- Get recommended cancer screenings.

- Take part in the health and safety committee.

- Follow the laboratory health and safety plan and learn about workplace hazards.

- Talk to your supervisor about any work-related concerns you have.

Summary

The numbers and types of cancer reported among employees of the CPD, CIS did not appear unusual and were unlikely related to workplace exposures. None of the chemicals used regularly were known to cause cancer in humans, and all personal exposures were below OELs. Recommendations were provided to correct problems with the design and function of the HVAC and LEV systems and to develop a forensic laboratory health and safety plan.

On November 18, 20, and 21, 2008, we conducted an HHE at the CPD, CIS. The HHE request, submitted by CPD management, concerned a possible cancer excess among former and current CIS employees. Other concerns listed in the request were IEQ, adequacy of the ventilation systems, chemical exposures encountered during criminal investigation procedures, and effectiveness of the engineering controls at minimizing chemical exposures in the crime lab. We obtained medical and employment information on current and former employees reported to have cancer. We verified their cancer types and employment duration in the CIS. We inspected all engineering controls, including the HVAC system, for deficiencies. We took measurements of CO_2 and airflow on the fourth, fifth, and sixth floors to evaluate the IEQ and performance of the HVAC system. We collected area air samples in the locations adjacent to the crime lab and photo-processing lab to evaluate the migration of chemicals throughout the building. We collected personal air samples for ethyl acetate during ninhydrin spraying, ethyl cyanoacrylate during super glue fuming, carbon black during fingerprint powder application, ammonia and sulfur dioxide during photo processing, and hydrogen peroxide during luminol spraying. We interviewed employees in a private setting to allow them to express their concerns and describe any symptoms related to their work.

The numbers and types of cancer reported among employees did not appear unusual, and the cancers were unlikely related to workplace exposures. Carbon black was the only chemical we identified that is used regularly and is listed by IARC as a possible human carcinogen. NIOSH considers carbon black carcinogenic only if it contains more than 0.1% PAHs. The carbon black used in the fingerprint powders did not contain measurable PAHs. Personal exposures to carbon black and all other chemicals evaluated in this survey were below applicable OELs.

The results of the area air sampling demonstrated the migration of ethyl acetate from the crime lab to other areas on the fifth floor. The super glue fuming chamber and associated filtration system controlled ethyl cyanoacrylate vapors inadequately. In addition to the crime lab, the photo-processing lab and bathrooms on the fourth and fifth floors were under positive pressure, which may allow contaminants and nuisance odors to move to other areas of the building. The evidence room was under slight negative pressure. However, because the evidence room did not have a dedicated exhaust system, the odor of the marijuana stored there as evidence was pungent inside and outside the room.

The fourth and fifth floors had multiple AHUs. Most of the outdoor air was delivered to the plenum (the space above the suspended ceiling) rather than ducted directly to the AHUs. These independently controlled AHUs likely contributed to the wide range of airflows (0–288 ft³/min) measured at the ceiling diffusers. Most of the HVAC air filters we inspected were dirty and needed to be replaced. In the afternoon (peak occupancy), CO_2 levels in the office areas on the fourth and fifth floors were greater than 700 ppm above the outdoor air levels (average of 425 ppm). This suggests that inadequate outdoor air was delivered to the office areas during peak occupancy.

Because ethyl cyanoacrylate vapors irritate the respiratory system and mucous membranes, we recommend replacing the super glue fuming chamber with a chamber that controls generated vapors more effectively. The HVAC system should be redesigned so that outdoor air is delivered to the AHUs and actively delivered to the occupied areas of the building. Filters in the HVAC system, fingerprint powder downdraft table, and small super glue fuming chamber should be replaced routinely. The ventilation system should be adjusted to maintain negative pressure in the crime lab, photo-processing lab, bathrooms, and other areas where contaminants and nuisance odors are generated. A dedicated exhaust system should be installed in the evidence room to control odors. A forensic laboratory health and safety plan should be developed. This plan should describe occupational hazards, standard operating procedures, engineering controls, and the PPE required for each method used to process criminal evidence.

Keywords: NAICS 922120 (Police Protection), crime lab, criminal investigation, forensics, latent fingerprint detection, fingerprint powder, carbon black, ninhydrin, luminol, ethyl acetate, ethyl cyanoacrylate, super glue fuming, indoor environmental quality, IEQ, cancer cluster, police

On July 18, 2008, NIOSH received a request from management at the CPD, CIS. The request concerned a possible excess of cancer among current and former employees. In addition, management expressed concern about chemical exposures encountered during criminal investigation procedures and about IEQ in the CIS on the fifth floor, as well as other areas of the building on the fourth, fifth, and sixth floors.

On November 18, 20, and 21, 2008, we conducted an HHE at the CPD, CIS. We met with management and employee representatives and observed work processes, practices, and workplace conditions. We were informed that five CIS employees had cancer. We obtained medical and employment information about the employees reported to have cancer. We interviewed employees privately to discuss their concerns and health symptoms they believed may be related to work. We collected area and personal air samples for chemicals used to process criminal evidence. We also evaluated the IEQ by inspecting the HVAC systems on the fourth, fifth, and sixth floors, and by measuring CO_2, airflow, and pressure differentials in several rooms throughout the building. A closing conference was held with management and employee representatives to summarize site visit activities and provide preliminary findings.

Workplace Description

The CPD, located at 824 Broadway Street in Cincinnati, Ohio, occupies the top three floors of a six-story building that was built in the 1920s as a newspaper warehouse. Each floor is approximately 6000 ft². The Major Offenders Unit, the Personal Crime Squad, and the Intelligence Section are on the fourth floor. The CIS and the Homicide Unit are on the fifth floor, and the evidence room occupies the entire sixth floor. Of the 101 CPD employees who work in the building, 21 are in the Major Offenders Unit, 24 in the Personal Crime Squad, 14 in the Intelligence Section, 5 in the evidence room, 21 in the Homicide Unit, and 16 in the CIS. Currently, the CIS consists of 14 criminalists who process criminal evidence (including 2 who work solely on video evidence) and 2 supervisory investigators. Since its inception in 1985, 47 officers have worked in the CIS.

The HVAC systems on the fourth, fifth, and sixth floors operated independently. The fourth and fifth floor HVAC systems consisted of multiple AHUs. Some of the AHUs were in the plenum (the space above the suspended ceiling), while others were in utility closets. Each AHU was controlled by a separate thermostat. Most of the outdoor air was actively drawn through fan-assisted air intakes on the side of the building and emptied into the plenum. A few air intakes passively provided outdoor air to the plenum without fan assistance. The sixth floor HVAC system had no outdoor air intake; thus, outdoor air entered by leaks through the building envelope (walls, windows, and ceiling) and was recirculated.

The crime lab (Figure 1) was on the fifth floor in the CIS. The crime lab was approximately 225 ft^2 and contained a fume hood for working with chemicals, a downdraft table for working with fingerprint powders, and two super glue fuming chambers. The large super glue fuming chamber vented to the outdoors, while the small fuming chamber had an organic vapor filtration system that vented to the indoors. The crime lab also contained an overhead exhaust hood for other work involving chemicals or dusts and a ninhydrin development cabinet that was not exhausted.

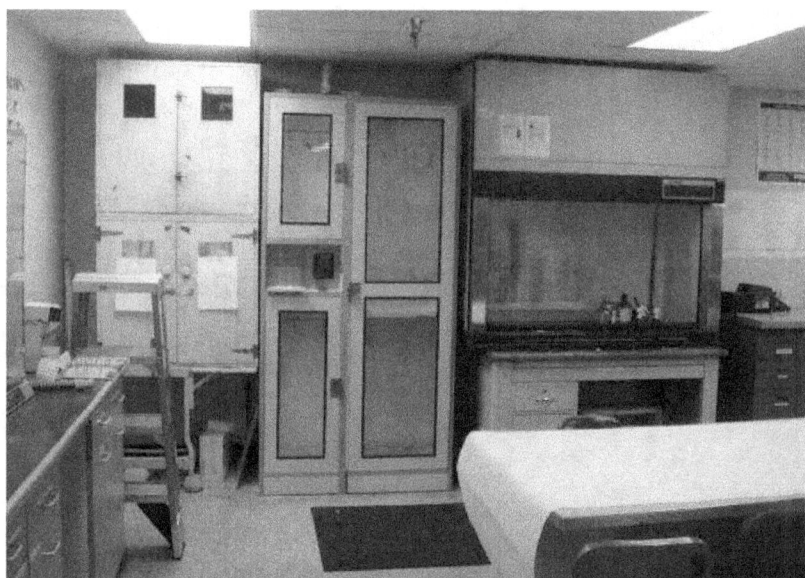

Figure 1. Ninhydrin development cabinet (left), large super glue fuming chamber (middle), and chemical fume hood (right) inside the crime lab.

A darkroom and photo processing lab (Figure 2) were adjacent to the crime lab. The darkroom, currently used for storage, contained an overhead exhaust hood. This hood used the same ventilation ductwork as the overhead exhaust hood in the crime lab. The photo processing lab did not contain a dedicated exhaust system but did contain an HVAC supply and return duct.

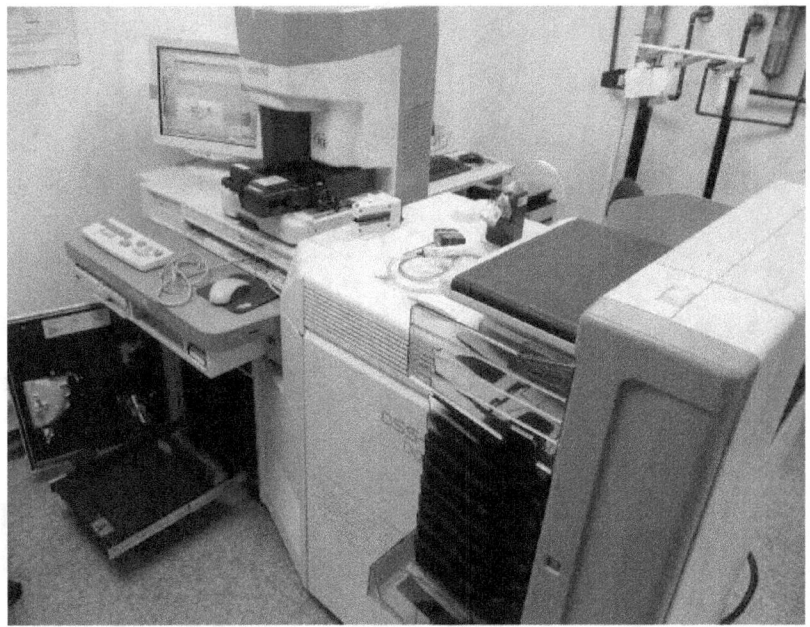

Figure 2. Photo printer inside the photo processing lab.

In addition to processing criminal evidence at the CPD, criminalists frequently go to a crime scene to gather and process evidence. During our investigation, criminalists did not go to a crime scene, but did go to the District 1 garage to apply fingerprint powder to an automobile involved in a crime. The District 1 garage was approximately 20 feet wide, 20 feet high, and 100 feet long.

Criminal Investigation Procedures

The CPD uses several methods for processing criminal evidence. Latent fingerprints are frequently identified using one of three methods: (1) fingerprint powder application, (2) ninhydrin solution spraying, and (3) super glue fuming. The black fingerprint powder used at the CPD contains carbon black. When the fingerprint powder is dusted over evidence or on surfaces at a crime scene, the carbon black adheres to residual oils fingers leave behind, thereby revealing ridge patterns or fingerprints. During our investigation, one criminalist applied the fingerprint powder to evidence using the downdraft table in the crime lab (Figure 3), and two criminalists applied the fingerprint powder to an automobile inside the District 1 garage (Figure 4). The criminalist who applied the fingerprint powder in the crime lab wore nitrile gloves and an N95 filtering facepiece respirator (AOSafety® Pleats Plus, 3M™, St. Paul, Minnesota). In the District 1 garage, one criminalist wore cloth coveralls, nitrile gloves, and a half-mask elastomeric respirator with type P100 particulate cartridges (Comfo Respirator, MSA®, Pittsburgh, Pennsylvania). The other criminalist wore Tyvek® coveralls (DuPont™, Wilmington, Delaware), nitrile gloves, and an AOSafety Pleats Plus N95 filtering facepiece respirator. All the garage doors were closed while the fingerprint powder was applied.

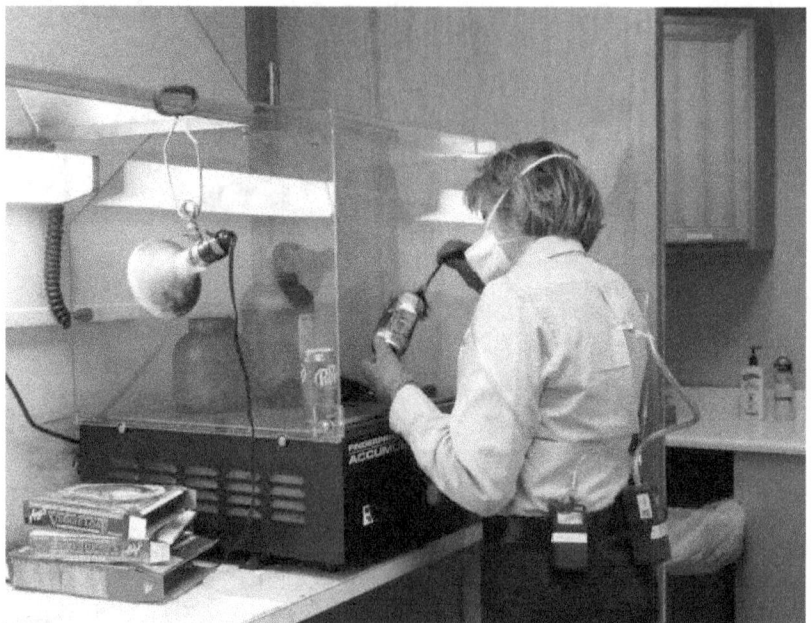

Figure 3. Application of black fingerprint powder to criminal evidence inside the enclosed downdraft table.

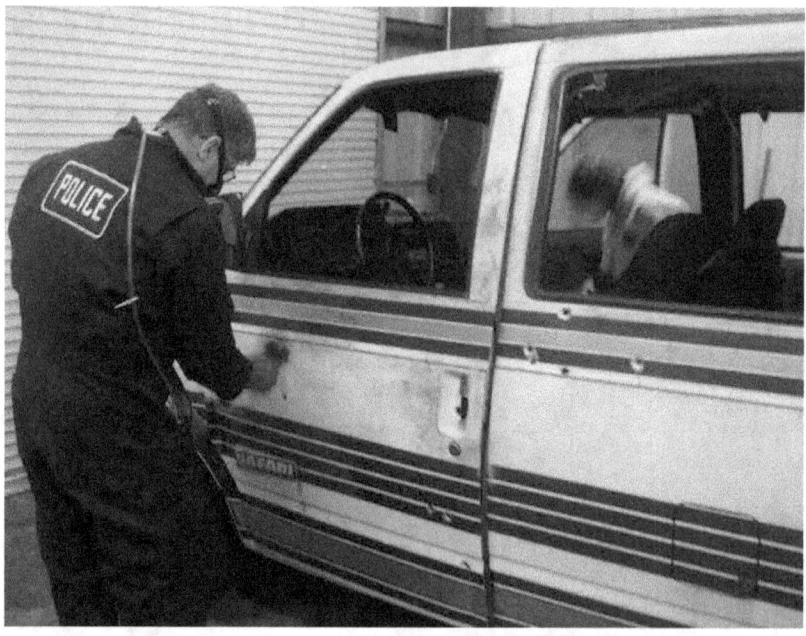

Figure 4. Application of black fingerprint powder to an automobile inside the District 1 garage.

Ninhydrin solution used by the CPD is made by mixing ethyl acetate, acetone, and dissolved ninhydrin powder crystals. When sprayed on evidence, the ninhydrin reacts with residual amino acids fingers leave behind to form a deep blue or purple fingerprint [Horswell 2004]. During our investigation, the ninhydrin solution was mixed just outside the chemical fume hood in the crime lab. After mixing, two criminalists sprayed ninhydrin solution on evidence under the chemical fume hood. After spraying and allowing time for the ninhydrin solution to dry, the evidence was transferred to the unventilated ninhydrin development cabinet (Figure 5). Both criminalists wore nitrile gloves, and one criminalist wore a half-mask respirator with combination organic vapor/ P95 filter cartridges (Dual Cartridge Respirator, 3M, St. Paul, Minnesota).

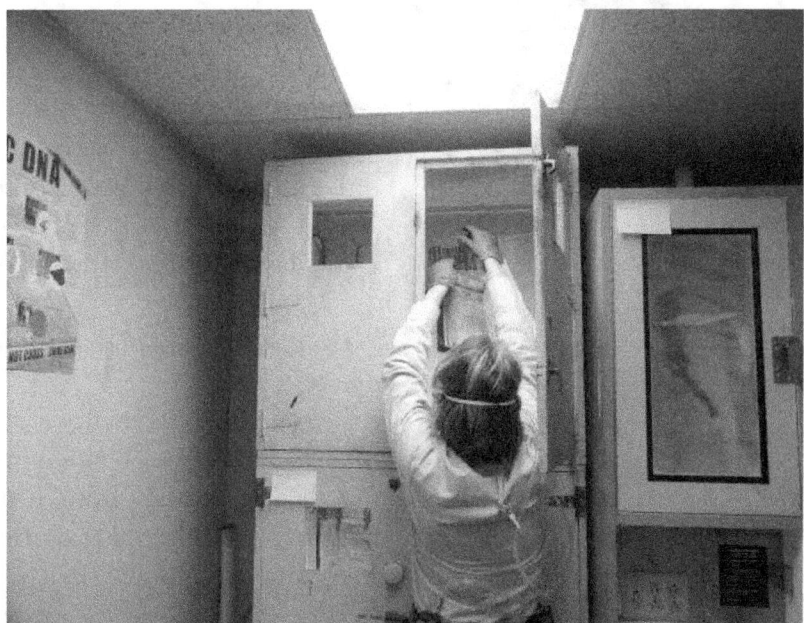

Figure 5. Transfer of criminal evidence previously sprayed with ninhydrin solution under the chemical fume hood to the ninhydrin development cabinet.

In the super glue fuming method, ethyl cyanoacrylate, the main ingredient in super glue, is heated inside a chamber containing evidence. The ethyl cyanoacrylate vapors and atmospheric moisture react with fingerprint residues to form a white polymer [Horswell 2004]. During our investigation, one criminalist used the small fuming chamber, and two criminalists used the large fuming chamber. The Plexiglas® doors of the fuming chambers were opened a few inches so the criminalists could view the progress of the fingerprint development (Figure 6) because the doors had become coated with super glue residue. The fuming chamber exhaust fans remained off during this time and were only turned

INTRODUCTION
(CONTINUED)

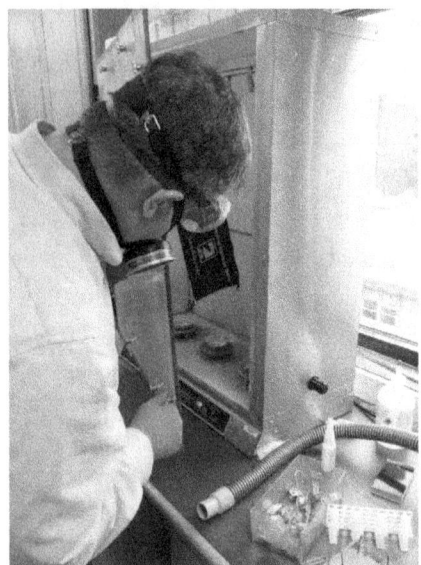

Figure 6. Criminalist opening the small super glue fuming chamber to view the fingerprint development.

on at the end of the fuming cycle to evacuate the chambers. All the criminalists wore nitrile gloves. Two criminalists wore MSA Comfo Respirators, and the other criminalist wore a 3M Dual Cartridge Respirator.

In addition to developing latent fingerprints, criminalists spray luminol solution for latent blood detection. When luminol solution is sprayed onto latent blood, the iron in the hemoglobin catalyzes the reaction between luminol and other components of the solution to produce chemiluminescence, which refers to the emission of light from a chemical reaction [Barni et al. 2007]. During our investigation, one criminalist wearing Tyvek coveralls and nitrile gloves sprayed the luminol solution onto mock evidence inside the District 1 garage.

Photo processing is another important duty for criminalists. Several chemicals are used to develop and print photographs, including ammonia and sodium bisulfite. Sulfur dioxide may be released during the thermal decomposition of sodium bisulfite [IPCS 1993]. During our investigation, one criminalist developed and printed photographs inside the photo processing lab adjacent to the crime lab. Nitrile gloves were worn when working with the chemicals.

ASSESSMENT

We obtained the names of the five CIS employees reported to have cancer. We obtained their employment history with the police department from the CIS and the CPD human resources office. Using information from medical records, death certificates obtained from CPD human resources, and one employee's spouse, we verified the cancer diagnosis for each employee. We reviewed the work materials used by employees to determine if any are known or suspected to cause cancer. We researched current medical information to determine if the types of cancers these employees had were known or suspected to be related to workplace exposures.

We interviewed CPD employees who worked in CIS, in the evidence room on the sixth floor, and on the fourth floor. These confidential interviews focused on medical, occupational, family, and social histories. This included, but was not limited to, work type and duration, past or current health conditions, medications, smoking status, possible workplace exposures, use of personal protective equipment, and work-related symptoms.

On November 18, 2008, we placed CO_2, temperature, and RH monitors in office areas on the fourth and fifth floors to assess the adequacy of the ventilation and its impact on the IEQ in these areas. These monitors are described in Appendix A. One monitor was placed in the middle of the Major Offenders Unit and Personal Crime Squad office areas on the fourth floor and CIS and in the Homicide Unit office areas on the fifth floor. On November 20, 2008, another monitor was placed in the evidence room on the sixth floor. All monitors operated until November 22, 2008.

On November 20, 2008, to further assess the IEQ, we evaluated the HVAC systems by inspecting the air filters in the AHUs and by measuring airflow through the supply and return ducts on the fourth and fifth floors. Using smoke tubes, we measured pressure differentials in rooms containing sources of chemicals or nuisance odors (i.e., crime lab, photo processing lab, evidence room, and bathrooms). We also used smoke tubes to qualitatively assess the capture efficiency of the LEV systems (i.e., chemical hood, downdraft table, overhead exhaust hoods, and super glue fuming chambers). In addition, we measured the air velocity through the LEV systems and inspected any filters in the LEV systems. The methods we used to evaluate the ventilation systems are described in Appendix A.

On November 21, 2008, we conducted both area and PBZ air sampling for chemicals used to process criminal evidence. Appendix B provides an overview of the chemicals used to process criminal evidence, including potential health effects and other important considerations for developing a sampling strategy. The OELs for the chemicals we sampled are presented in Table 1. The air sampling methods we used are described in Appendix A. Area air sampling was performed inside the crime lab and in areas adjacent to the crime lab for the entire work shift (approximately 8 hours). Figure C1 (Appendix C) provides a schematic of the area air sampling locations and chemicals that were measured at each location.

Table 1. Occupational exposure limits for chemicals used to process criminal evidence at the CPD.

	Ethyl acetate (ppm)	Ethyl cyanoacrylate (ppm)	Sulfur dioxide (ppm)	Ammonia (ppm)	Hydrogen peroxide (ppm)	Carbon black (mg/m³)
OSHA PEL	400	N/A*	5	50	1	3.5
NIOSH REL	400	N/A*	2	25	1	3.5†
ACGIH TLV	400	0.2	2	25	1	3.5

* N/A = not applicable
† If carbon black contains PAHs, the NIOSH REL is 0.1 mg/m³.

The PBZ air samples were collected during specific tasks. Some tasks lasted a few minutes (e.g., ninhydrin spraying), and other tasks lasted the entire work shift (e.g., photo processing). We collected two PBZ samples of ethyl acetate during ninhydrin solution spraying and three PBZ samples of ethyl cyanoacrylate during super glue fuming. We collected one PBZ sample of carbon black during the application of fingerprint dust on evidence inside the crime lab and two PBZ samples of carbon black during the application of fingerprint dust on an automobile inside the District 1 garage. A bulk sample of the black fingerprint powder was collected for the analysis of PAHs. We collected one PBZ sample for ammonia and one PBZ sample for sulfur dioxide during photo processing. We collected two colorimetric indicator tube samples for hydrogen peroxide in the headspace of the luminol solution spray bottle. Because luminol solution contains sodium carbonate, we also measured its alkalinity using pH paper.

RESULTS

Cancer

The five employees reported to have cancer each had a different type of cancer: lung adenocarcinoma, bile duct cholangiocarcinoma, multiple myeloma, melanoma, and non-Hodgkin lymphoma. They were diagnosed between 1998 and 2008. Four were deceased; the average age at death was 62 years. The employee still living was currently not working because of his illness. Their average duration of employment in the CIS was 16 years. Four were smokers and one never smoked.

Employee Interviews

We interviewed 13 employees: 6 Criminalists, 3 Personal Crimes Detectives, 2 Evidence Room workers, 1 Polygraph Examiner, and 1 Intelligence Officer. The employees' average age was 44.6 years. Their average duration of employment in the building was 5 years, ranging from 8 months to 23 years. Two employees were current smokers; three were former smokers; and eight never smoked. Of the 13 employees interviewed, four reported they had no symptoms related to working in the building. One employee in Personal Crimes reported having migraines but was not sure if they were worse since starting work in the building. Eight employees reported work-related health symptoms. Three CIS employees had complaints: one described headaches, one described headaches and tingling around the face when using ninhydrin, and one complained of a hacking cough that had lasted one year. Two Evidence Room employees had complaints: one described a cough and hoarse voice that was worse on Mondays and better over the weekend, and a "brain fog" that improved when away from the work area; one complained of nasal congestion and sneezing. Two Personal Crimes Detectives had complaints: one described seasonal allergies that improved when off work, loss of voice, productive cough, headache, and constant drainage; one described allergies, congestion, raspy voice, and itchy, watery eyes that began when entering the building. A Polygraph Examiner complained of a headache, shortness of breath, and red itchy eyes that improved when not in the building, and needing to use albuterol since starting work at CPD.

Indoor Environmental Quality and Ventilation Assessment

Table 2 summarizes the CO_2, temperature, and RH measurements collected over time in office areas on the fourth and fifth floors and in the evidence room on the sixth floor. Figures C2, C3, and C4 in Appendix C illustrate the trend in CO_2 levels over time for these areas. In general, CO_2 levels were the highest in the afternoon (>1000 ppm for the fourth and fifth floor office areas) and lowest in the early morning. Airflow measurements taken at the supply diffusers and return grilles on the fourth and fifth floors ranged from 0 to 280 ft³/min. We stopped collecting these measurements when it became apparent that the HVAC systems on the fourth and fifth floors were composed of several independently-controlled AHUs. The measurements we did collect demonstrated that the airflow varied greatly throughout these two floors and depended on the thermostat settings (auto, on, off). The ventilation smoke tube measurements indicated that the crime lab, photo processing lab, and bathrooms on the fifth floor were all under positive pressure in relation to the surrounding areas.

Table 2. Summary of CO_2, temperature, and RH measurements on the fourth, fifth, and sixth floors.

Office space location	Sampling time (hrs)	CO_2 (ppm)		Temp (°F)		RH (%)	
		Range	Mean	Range	Mean	Range	Mean
Fourth floor Major Offenders Unit	94	540 – 2010	1020	68 – 74	70	19 – 38	25
Fourth floor Personal Crime Squad	94	430 – 1650	860	71 – 80	76	16 – 33	18
Fifth floor CIS	94	450 – 1600	790	71 – 75	74	18 – 33	22
Fifth floor Homicide Unit	94	440 – 1400	750	74 – 77	75	18 – 28	19
Sixth floor Evidence Room	50	420 – 720	560	73 – 75	73	18 – 22	21

Most of the filters in the AHUs of the HVAC systems on the fourth and fifth floors were dirty and needed immediate replacement. Several filters were pieced together using roll-type low-efficiency prefilter material (Figure 7), rather than properly sized and framed higher efficiency filters. The downdraft table in the crime lab had a prefilter and high-efficiency filter. Visual assessment revealed that most of the fingerprint powder was collected by the prefilter. The high-efficiency filter had not been changed in 9 years and showed visible evidence of breakthrough (fingerprint powder on the back of the filter). The small super glue fuming chamber contained an organic vapor filtration system consisting of a prefilter and activated-carbon filter. Neither filter had been changed in several months. We could smell ethyl cyanoacrylate vapors coming through the filtration system during the super glue fuming operation, suggesting either that the activated carbon filter had become saturated with ethyl cyanoacrylate vapors or that there was leakage around the filter.

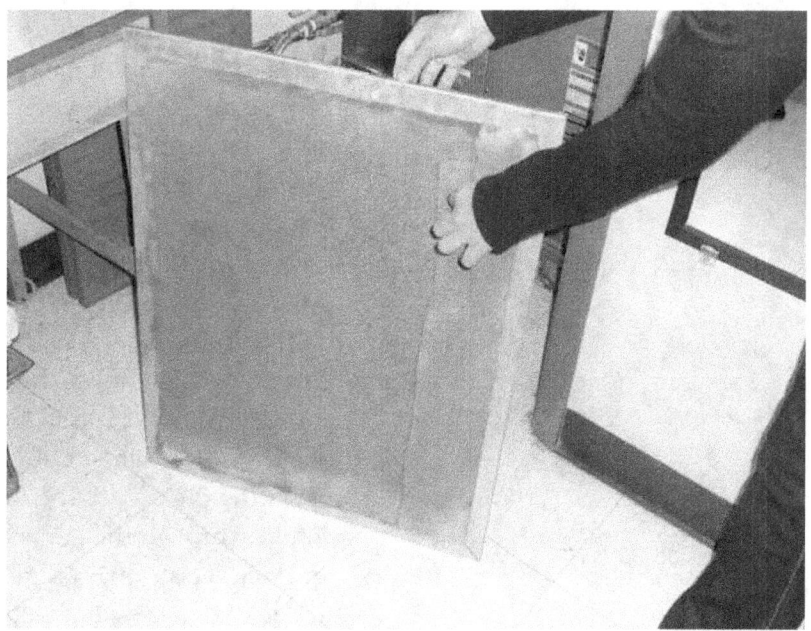

Figure 7. Dirty air filter removed from the HVAC system made of pieces of roll-type low-efficiency prefilter material.

The area air sampling results are summarized in Table 3. The area sampling results show the migration of ethyl acetate from the crime lab to other areas of the building. Ethyl cyanoacrylate vapors were detected in the crime lab, but not in areas adjacent to the crime lab. All other area sampling results were ND, defined as concentrations below the MDC of 0.004 ppm for ethyl cyanoacrylate, 0.0002 ppm for sulfur dioxide, and 0.15 ppm for ammonia. These concentrations are well below applicable OELs.

Table 3. Summary of the area air sampling results.

Location	Ethyl acetate (ppm)	Ethyl cyanoacrylate (ppm)*	Sulfur dioxide (ppm)[†]	Ammonia (ppm)[‡]
Crime lab	0.30	(0.008)	Not sampled	Not sampled
Criminalist office area	0.14	ND	Not sampled	Not sampled
Outside crime lab, next to photo tables	0.14	ND	Not sampled	Not sampled
Photo processing lab	Not sampled	Not sampled	ND	ND
Video evidence area	0.09	ND	ND	ND

* Values in parentheses represent trace concentrations below the MQC (0.046 ppm) but above the MDC (0.004 ppm).
[†] The MDC was 0.0002 ppm.
[‡] The MDC was 0.15 ppm.

RESULTS
(CONTINUED)

Table 4 summarizes the air velocity measurements and smoke tube testing on the LEV systems used in the CIS. The average air velocity for the LEV systems ranged from 2.5 ft/min for the small fuming chamber with the door open 1 inch to 89 ft/min for the chemical fume hood with the sash half opened. Smoke tube testing demonstrated effective capture of smoke for all the LEV systems except the overhead hoods and super glue fuming chambers when the doors were opened 1 inch. Smoke tube testing for the overhead hoods was performed at the work stations approximately 4 feet below the hoods. Slight turbulence was observed for the chemical hood near the bottom of the sash at fully opened and half opened sash heights. Using smoke tubes, we also found that when operating the exhaust hood in the crime lab, air could be detected coming through the darkroom exhaust hood (when turned off), and vice versa. This "backflow" of air occurred because these two hoods shared the same ductwork.

Table 4. Evaluation of the LEV systems used in the CIS.*

Type of LEV system	Area of face (ft²)	Air velocity (ft/min)		Effective capture of smoke?
		Range	Mean	
Chemical fume hood (fully opened sash)	9.4	36 – 70	57	Yes
Chemical fume hood (half opened sash)	4.7	37 – 160	89	Yes
Fingerprint powder (enclosed downdraft table)	3.0	40 – 90	62	Yes
Large super glue fuming chamber (closed door/open baffle)	0.3	500 – 540	520	Yes
Large super glue fuming chamber (door opened one inch)	6.5	5 – 25	15	No
Small super glue fuming chamber (closed door/open baffle)	0.3	100 – 110	107	Yes
Small super glue fuming chamber (door opened one inch)	2.6	1 – 4	2.5	No
Overhead exhaust hood (crime lab)[†]	6.7	13 – 120	72	No
Overhead exhaust hood (darkroom)[‡]	6.7	52 – 82	67	No

* Air velocity measurements were taken at the face or opening where air was being drawn, while smoke tube testing was conducted at the work area where contaminants were being captured or contained.
[†] The mean capture velocity at the work area (4 feet below the hood) was 3 ft/min.
[‡] The mean capture velocity at the work area (4 feet below the hood) was 1.6 ft/min.

Personal Breathing Zone Sampling

The PBZ sampling results are provided in Table 5 for ethyl acetate, Table 6 for ethyl cyanoacrylate, and Table 7 for carbon black. All PBZ concentrations were below applicable OELs. The black fingerprint powder did not contain PAHs. Ammonia concentrations were ND (below the MDC of 0.16 ppm). Likewise, sulfur dioxide concentrations were ND (below the MDC of 0.00081 ppm). All PBZ results were well below applicable OELs. Hydrogen peroxide was ND in the headspace of the luminol solution spray bottle and the luminol solution was basic (pH = 11).

Table 5. PBZ sampling results for ethyl acetate during ninhydrin spraying.

Process location	Process description	Sampling time (min)	Concentration (ppm)	OEL* (ppm)
Chemical fume hood and table inside the crime lab	Spraying and mixing	170	0.92	400
Chemical fume hood	Spraying	14	13	400

* Refers to NIOSH REL, OSHA PEL, and ACGIH TLV for ethyl acetate.

Table 6. PBZ sampling results for ethyl cyanoacrylate during super glue fuming.

Process location	Process description	Sampling time (min)	Concentration (ppm)	OEL* (ppm)
Large fuming chamber	Developing fingerprints	169	ND[†]	0.2
Large fuming chamber	Developing fingerprints	143	ND[†]	0.2
Small fuming chamber	Developing fingerprints	199	0.022	0.2

* Refers to ACGIH TLV; NIOSH and OSHA do not have OELs for ethyl cyanoacrylate.
[†] ND = concentration is below the MDC of 0.014 ppm.

RESULTS
(CONTINUED)

Table 7. PBZ sampling results for carbon black during black fingerprint powder application.

Process location	Process description	Sampling time (min)	Concentration (mg/m³)*	OEL‡ (mg/m³)
Downdraft table	Applying fingerprint powder to evidence	120	ND	3.5
District 1 garage	Applying fingerprint powder to a car	30	(0.88)†	3.5
District 1 garage	Applying fingerprint powder to a car	31	2.3	3.5

* ND = concentration is below the MDC of 0.48 mg/m³
† Values in parentheses represent concentrations above the MDC of 0.48 mg/m³ and below MQC of 1.49 mg/m³.
‡ Refers to NIOSH REL, OSHA PEL, and ACGIH TLV for ethyl acetate.

DISCUSSION

Cancer Clusters

Because of the concerns among the CIS employees about cancer, it is helpful to review some general information about cancer, and the approach we take in determining whether cancers have any relationship to the workplace.

Cancer is a group of different diseases that have the same feature: the uncontrolled growth and spread of abnormal cells. Each different type of cancer may have its own set of causes. Cancer is common in the United States. Approximately 1,479,390 men and women will be diagnosed with cancer and 562,340 will die of cancer in all sites in 2009 [National Cancer Institute 2009]. One of every four deaths in the United States is from cancer. Among adults, cancer is more frequent among men than women, and is more frequent with increasing age. Many factors play a role in the development of cancer. The importance of these factors is different for different types of cancer. Most cancers are caused by a combination of several factors. Some of the factors include (1) personal characteristics such as age, sex, and race; (2) family history of cancer; (3) diet; (4) personal habits such as cigarette smoking and alcohol consumption; (5) the presence of certain medical conditions; (6) exposure to cancer causing agents in the environment; and (7) exposure to cancer causing agents in the workplace. In many cases, these factors may act together or in sequence to cause cancer. Although some causes of some types of cancer are known, we don't know everything about the causes of cancer [American Cancer Society 2009].

DISCUSSION
(CONTINUED)

Cancers often appear to occur in clusters, which scientists define as an unusual concentration of cancer cases in a defined area or time [CDC 1990]. A cluster also occurs when the cancers are found among employees of a different age or sex group than is usual. The cases of cancer may have a common cause or may be the coincidental occurrence of unrelated causes. The number of cases may seem high, particularly among a small group of people who have something in common with the cases, such as working in the same building. Although the occurrence of a disease may be random, diseases often are not distributed randomly in the population, and clusters of disease may arise by chance alone [Metz and McGuinness 1997]. In many workplaces the number of cases is small. This makes detecting whether the cases have a common cause difficult, especially when there are no apparent cancer-causing exposures. It is common for the borders of the perceived cluster to be drawn where the cases of cancer are located, instead of defining the population and geographic area first. This often leads to the inaccurate belief that the rate of cancer is high.

When cancer in a workplace is described, it is important to learn whether the type of cancer is a primary cancer or a metastasis (spread of the primary cancer into other organs). Only primary cancers are used to investigate a cancer cluster. To assess whether the cancers among employees could be related to occupational exposures, we consider the number of cancer cases, the types of cancer, the likelihood of exposures to potential cancer-causing agents, and the timing of the diagnosis of cancer in relation to the exposure. These issues are discussed below as they relate to the request.

Do more CIS employees have cancer than people who do not work in the CIS?

Because cancer is a common disease, it may be found among people at any workplace. In the United States, one in two men and one in three women will develop cancer over the course of their lifetimes [American Cancer Society 2009]. These numbers do not include basal or squamous cell skin cancers, which are very common (over 1 million diagnosed annually), or any in situ carcinomas other than bladder. (In situ refers to cancer that has not yet spread beyond where it began; it is considered a precursor form of cancer.) If these were included, rates would be even higher. When several cases of cancer occur in a workplace they may be part of a true cluster when the number is greater than we expect compared to other groups of people similar in age, sex, and race. Disease or tumor rates, however, are highly variable in small populations and rarely match the overall rate for a larger area, such as the state, so that for any given time period some populations have rates above the overall rate and other have rates below the overall rate. So, even when an excess occurs, this may be completely consistent with the expected random variability. In addition, calculations like this make many assumptions that may not be appropriate for every workplace. Comparing rates without adjusting for age, sex, or other population characteristics assumes that such characteristics are the same in the workplace as in the larger population, which may not be true. However, general information on cancer rates is useful for providing perspective on the cancers in your population. Five cases of cancer in a 10-year span among 47 employees do not appear excessive.

Does the CPD have an unusual distribution of types of cancer?

Cancer clusters thought to be related to a workplace exposure usually consist of the same types of cancer. When several cases of the same type of cancer occur and that type is not common in the general population, it is more likely that an occupational exposure is involved. When the cluster consists of multiple types of cancer, without one type predominating, then an occupational cause of the cluster is less likely. The five officers with cancer each had a different type of cancer. This suggests lack of a common exposure and that an occupational cause of their cancers is unlikely.

Is exposure to a specific chemical or physical agent known or suspected of causing cancer occurring?

The relationship between some agents and certain cancers has been well established. With other agents and cancers the relationship is suspected, but the evidence is not definitive. When a known or suspected cancer-causing agent is present and the types of cancer occurring have been linked with these exposures in other settings, we are more likely to make the connection between cancer and a workplace exposure. None of the chemicals used regularly in CIS were known to be carcinogenic to humans.

Has enough time passed since exposure began?

The time between first exposure to a cancer-causing agent and clinical recognition of the disease is called the latency period. Latency periods vary by cancer type, but usually are a minimum of 10–12 years [Rugo 2004]. For example, it can take up to 30 years after exposure to asbestos for mesothelioma to develop. Because of this, past exposures are more relevant than current exposures as potential causes of cancers occurring in employees today. One employee worked in the CIS for only 2 years before he was diagnosed with cancer, making it extremely unlikely that the cancer was associated with working in CIS. The other four worked in CIS an average of 16 years, ranging from 12 to 23 years. However, we did not find an excess of cancer or any significant hazardous exposures in the CIS; therefore, latency is not pertinent in this evaluation.

Work Related Symptoms

Most symptoms (cough, itchy eyes, sneezing, hoarse voice, nasal congestion, headache, allergies, "brain fog," face tingling) reported by employees are common in buildings with poor IEQ. However, these symptoms are nonspecific and can also have many nonoccupational causes. We were not able to identify any single cause of these symptoms, but we did identify a variety of issues that can be addressed to improve the overall IEQ in the CPD building.

Chemical Exposures

All area and PBZ sampling results were below applicable OELs and therefore represent conditions under which nearly all employees may be exposed over a working lifetime without adverse health effects [ACGIH 2009]. However, the PBZ concentrations measured during the application of carbon black fingerprint powder to a car approached the OEL of 3 5 mg/m^3, suggesting that criminalists' exposure to carbon black to may approach the OEL if this activity was done over an entire workday (8 hours). Thus, we cannot say with confidence that exposures to carbon black during crime scene processing do not exceed the OEL on some days.

Indoor Environmental Quality

One of the most common deficiencies in the indoor environment is the improper operation and maintenance of ventilation systems and other building components [NIOSH 1991]. NIOSH investigators have found that correcting HVAC problems often reduces reported symptoms. For example, improving HVAC operation and maintenance, increasing ventilation rates, and maintaining comfortable temperature and RH can all potentially serve to improve symptoms without ever identifying any specific cause-effect relationships. When conducting an IEQ survey, we often measure ventilation and comfort indicators, such as CO_2, temperature, and RH to provide information relative to the functioning and control of HVAC systems.

According to Appendix C of the ANSI/ASHRAE Standard 62.1-2007, CO_2 levels in the indoor air should be maintained at a steady state no greater than about 700 ppm above outdoor air levels [ASHRAE 2007a]. During this evaluation, CO_2 levels in the fourth and fifth floor offices gradually increased throughout the morning to levels in the afternoon that were above this guideline (see Figures C2, C3, and C4 in Appendix C). A normal constituent of exhaled breath, CO_2 is not considered a building air pollutant. However, elevated CO_2 concentrations suggest that other indoor contaminants may also be increased. If CO_2 concentrations are elevated, the amount of outdoor air introduced into the ventilated space may need to be increased. ANSI/ASHRAE Standard 62.1-2007 recommends outdoor air supply rates of 17 ft^3/min/person for office spaces and libraries and 7 ft^3/min/person for reception areas [ASHRAE 2007a].

Temperature and RH did not vary greatly over time in the office areas on the fourth and fifth floors and in the evidence room on the sixth floor (see Table 2). The greatest swing in temperature (71°F–80°F) was observed in the Personal Crime Squad office area, most likely because of changes in the thermostat setting. As a result, on more than one occasion, the temperature and RH in the Personal Crime Squad office area were above the acceptable range of operative temperature and humidity for thermal comfort as specified in ANSI/ASHRAE Standard 55-2004 [ASHRAE 2004]. The temperature and RH measured in the other areas of the building were within the acceptable range.

DISCUSSION

Several rooms having potential sources of nuisance odors (i.e., bathrooms, photo processing lab, and crime lab) were under positive pressure in relation to surrounding areas, suggesting that these nuisance odors could flow from these rooms and into adjacent offices. This is one explanation why ethyl acetate vapors were detected in rooms adjacent to the crime lab. Although the evidence room on the sixth floor was under slight negative pressure relative to the entryway and stairway surrounding the room, the absence of a dedicated exhaust system allowed marijuana odors to accumulate in this area and eventually travel to other areas of the building. For example, we found that the elevators functioned much like pistons, pulling marijuana odors from the sixth floor evidence room down into the fifth and fourth floors.

ASHRAE recommends minimum exhaust rates of 50 ft³/min per toilet or urinal for bathrooms, 1.0 ft³/min per square foot for darkrooms [ASHRAE 2007a], and six air changes per hour for occupied laboratories [ASHRAE 2007b]. Although no specific recommendations are provided by ASHRAE for evidence rooms, the recommended exhaust rate for occupied laboratories of six air changes per hour has been used in the past as a guideline for evidence rooms [NIOSH 1999].

Several air filters examined in the HVAC systems, as well as the LEV systems in the crime lab, were dirty and needed immediate replacement (see Figure 7). Dirty filters increase the back-pressure on the ventilation system and potentially decrease the amount of air delivered to the occupied spaces (for HVAC systems) or decrease the amount of air that is exhausted (for LEV systems). Similarly, the organic vapor filters like the one used in the small super glue fuming chamber should be changed according to manufacturer's recommendations. Otherwise the activated carbon in the organic vapor filters can become saturated over time and lose the ability to collect organic vapors. This is likely why ethyl cyanoacrylate vapors were detected in the exhaust stream of the small super glue fuming chamber. Finally, we observed air filters in several HVAC systems that consisted of a combination of several loose sections of filter material that did not fit tightly within the filter frame. This could allow unfiltered air to leak around the sides of the filters.

ASHRAE provides recommendations and guidance for the evaluation of laboratory LEV systems [ASHRAE 2007b]. Generally, ASHRAE does not specify air velocity rates for LEV systems. Instead, they rely largely on visualization methods and tracer gas tests to ensure that contaminants are being captured. Smoke tube testing is one simple way of evaluating the capture efficiency of LEV systems for gases and vapors. The smoke we generated was not captured efficiently by the overhead exhaust hoods or by the super glue fuming chambers when their doors were opened 1 inch.

The overhead exhaust hoods were used sparingly during our investigation. For example, magnetic fingerprint powders containing iron were used under the overhead exhaust hood in the crime lab by one criminalist, and this procedure lasted only a few minutes. Nevertheless, because the overhead exhaust hoods in the crime lab and darkroom shared the same ductwork, the potential exists for contaminants to be exhausted from one hood to the other hood.

The super glue fuming chambers were used by three different criminalists at various times throughout the workday. The Plexiglas doors of the fuming chambers were opened a few inches so the criminalists could view the progress of the fingerprint development (see Figure 6). The exhaust fans remained off during this time but even if they had been turned on, our findings suggest that the air velocity would be inadequate to efficiently capture ethyl cyanoacrylate vapors. This is probably another reason why we measured detectable concentrations of ethyl cyanoacrylate vapors in the crime lab.

The ANSI/American Industrial Hygiene Association Standard Z9.5-2003 specifies that most chemical fume hoods can be operated effectively at 80–100 ft/min; however, operating chemical fume hoods below 60 ft/min is not recommended [AIHA 2003]. The air velocity we measured through the chemical fume hood was below the minimum level when the sash was fully opened (57 ft/min) but within the recommended range when the sash was half opened (89 ft/min). The hood was operated at both sash heights during our evaluation. According to our smoke tube testing, the chemical fume hood was efficiently capturing contaminants at both sash heights. Nevertheless, keeping the sash at half opened height or lower during use should improve the capture efficiency. Irrespective of the chemical fume hood capture efficiency, the most likely causes for detectable concentrations of ethyl acetate in the crime lab were that the criminalists mixed ninhydrin solution outside the chemical fume hood and transferred the sprayed evidence to the development cabinets before the evidence had completely dried.

CONCLUSIONS

It is unlikely that the reported cancers are associated with working in the CIS. This conclusion is based on the following:

- The number and types of cancers do not appear unusual.
- The different types of cancers do not suggest a common exposure.
- No significant hazardous exposures were identified.

PBZ air sampling identified no exposures to any chemicals used in CIS that were over OELs. Nevertheless, an opportunity exists for improving work conditions and overall IEQ. Our findings suggest inadequacies with the HVAC systems on the fourth, fifth, and sixth floors; super glue fuming chambers; and overhead exhaust hoods currently being used at the CPD. Exhaust ventilation was absent or insufficient in rooms containing sources of contaminants or nuisance odors.

RECOMMENDATIONS

We do not recommend any further investigation of cancer among CIS employees. Although the reported cases of cancers were not likely due to a workplace exposure, employees may have concerns about their own risk for cancer. Therefore, we recommend encouraging employees to learn about the following:

- Known cancer risk factors
- Measures to reduce risk for preventable cancers
- Availability of cancer screening programs for certain types of cancer

The following internet resources may be useful in addressing concerns:

- American Cancer Society website at www.cancer.org
- National Cancer Institute website at www.cancer.gov
- NIOSH occupational cancer and cancer cluster investigations topic page at www.cdc.gov/niosh/topics/cancer/

RECOMMENDATIONS
(CONTINUED)

Employees can take an active role in changing personal risk factors that are associated with certain types of cancer. In fact, the American Cancer Society estimates that half of all cancer deaths in the United States were preventable [American Cancer Society 2009]. In 2006, tobacco use alone caused an estimated 168,000 cancer deaths. It is well known that tobacco use is the single largest preventable cause of disease and increases the risk of 13 cancers: lung, mouth, nasal cavities, larynx, pharynx, esophagus, stomach, liver, pancreas, kidney, bladder, uterine cervix, and myeloid leukemia. High alcohol consumption, a diet low in fruits and vegetables, physical inactivity, overweight, and obesity are other modifiable personal risk factors that increase the risk of certain cancers. In fact, approximately one third of all cancer deaths in 2007 were related to poor nutrition, physical inactivity, and a high body mass index (BMI, a relationship between weight and height associated with body fat and health risk). Abundant scientific evidence shows that higher levels of BMI are associated with an increased risk of 15 types of cancer: esophagus, stomach, colorectal, liver, gallbladder, pancreas, prostate, kidney, non-Hodgkin lymphoma, multiple myeloma, leukemia, breast, uterus, cervix, and ovary.

Another significant way for employees to prevent morbidity and mortality from cancer is to get cancer screening tests recommended for persons of their age and/or sex (i.e., colonoscopies for colon cancer screening, mammograms for breast cancer screening). Employees need to discuss available cancer screening programs with their primary care physicians. This can lead to earlier detection of cancers and earlier treatment that may increase the chances of curing the disease.

Based on our other findings, we recommend the actions listed below to create a more healthful workplace. We encourage the CPD, CIS to use these recommendations to develop an action plan based, if possible, on the hierarchy of controls approach (refer to Appendix B). This approach groups actions by their likely effectiveness in reducing or removing hazards. In most cases, the preferred approach is to eliminate hazardous materials or processes and install engineering controls to reduce exposure or shield employees. Until such controls are in place, or if they are not effective or feasible, administrative measures and/or personal protective equipment may be needed.

Engineering Controls

Engineering controls reduce employees' exposures by removing the hazard from the process or placing a barrier between the hazard and the employee. Engineering controls are very effective at protecting employees without placing primary responsibility of implementation on the employee.

1. Further evaluate the HVAC systems on the fourth, fifth, and sixth floors to determine the best approach to ensure that an adequate amount of outdoor air is delivered to the occupied workspaces. Refer to ANSI/ASHRAE Standard 62.1-2007 for guidance [ASHRAE 2007a]. We were unable to pinpoint the primary reason for the inadequate amount of outdoor air supply because the HVAC systems were made up of several AHUs that were controlled by separate thermostats set to different settings (auto, on, off). Ideally, outdoor air intakes should be ducted to the AHUs rather than emptying to the plenum, each HVAC system should have a single AHU that operates continuously, and thermostats should be set to temperatures within the acceptable range for the humidity level as specified in ANSI/ASHRAE Standard 55-2004 [ASHRAE 2004]. This arrangement would allow greater control of the outdoor air supply, airflow, and thermal comfort levels throughout the different floors of the building.

2. Replace air filters routinely. Filters used in the HVAC system and prefilters used in the fingerprint powder downdraft table should be replaced at least every 3 months with properly sized filters rated per the manufacturer specifications. According to manufacturer specifications (Payton Scientific, Buffalo, New York), the high efficiency filter in the fingerprint powder downdraft table should be replaced every 4–6 months in a busy laboratory. The pressure gauge can also be used to determine when the filter should be replaced [Fingerprint Powder Accumulator 2005].

3. Maintain the crime lab, photo processing lab, evidence room, bathrooms, and other rooms with potential sources of contaminants or nuisance odors under negative pressure relative to the adjacent areas. Specific guidance on appropriate exhaust rates is provided in ANSI/ASHRAE Standard 62.1-2007 [ASHRAE 2007a] and Chapter 14 of the ASHRAE Handbook [ASHRAE 2007b].

4. Increase the airflow through the overhead exhaust hoods to ensure efficient capture velocity. Under their current design, these hoods should only be used for processes involving volatile or semivolatile chemicals that cannot otherwise be performed under the chemical fume hood (e.g., objects that are too big for the fume hood). These hoods should not be used for fingerprint powder application as the upward airflow could actually draw the dust into the criminalists' PBZs. The downdraft table or a new slot hood would better control the fingerprint powder.

5. Install separate ductwork for each of the overhead exhaust hoods. Alternatively, cap or remove the exhaust hood in the dark room or operate both hoods at the same time. Because they currently share the same ductwork, contaminants exhausted from the darkroom could be entrained into the crime lab (when the crime lab hood is shut off) and vice versa.

6. Begin to replace super glue fuming chambers with ones that have the following safety features: (1) glass window enclosures with locking mechanisms that cannot be opened during use until the chambers are fully evacuated, (2) exhaust systems that vent to the outdoors and/or contain organic vapor filtration systems, (3) laboratory determined filter change out schedule based on number of cycles or end of service life indicator, and (4) counters that display the number of cycles run since last filter change out.

Administrative Controls

Administrative controls are management dictated work practices and policies to reduce or prevent exposures to workplace hazards. The effectiveness of administrative changes in work practices for controlling workplace hazards is dependent on management commitment and employee acceptance. Regular monitoring and reinforcement is necessary to ensure that control policies and procedures are not circumvented in the name of convenience or production.

1. Reduce criminalists' exposures to chemicals by only handling chemicals (pouring, mixing, spraying, etc.) under the chemical fume hood. Evidence sprayed with ninhydrin solution should be allowed to dry completely before being placed into the development cabinet.

2. Have the chemical fume hood tested and certified annually. The sash of the chemical fume hood should be maintained at half opened height or lower during use to further improve its performance. Marking the half opened height will serve as a reminder to operate the fume hood at that height.

3. Develop a written forensic laboratory health and safety plan that describes workplace hazards, standard operating procedures, engineering controls, and PPE required for each method criminalists use to process evidence at the CPD. For guidance, refer to the International Association for Identification, *Safety Guidelines* [IAI 2004] and the Federal Bureau of Investigation, *Handbook of Forensic Services* [FBI 2007]. This plan should be updated regularly (e.g., annually) or as needed.

4. Organize a health and safety committee consisting of management and employee representatives who meet regularly to address health and safety concerns and update the laboratory health and safety plan.

5. Collect additional air samples for carbon black during the application of black fingerprint powder at a crime scene. Several samples (> three) should be collected over 8 hours during representative crime scene processing to obtain a more accurate estimate of the average PBZ concentration over an entire shift and variability around this estimate. This will provide greater confidence that exposures are above or below the OEL of 3.5 mg/m^3.

Personal Protective Equipment

PPE is the least effective means for controlling employee exposures. Proper use of PPE requires a comprehensive program and calls for a high level of employee involvement and commitment to be effective. Using PPE requires the choice of the appropriate equipment to reduce the hazard and the development of supporting programs such as training, change-out schedules, and medical assessment if needed. PPE should not be relied upon as the sole method for limiting employee exposures. Rather, PPE should be used until engineering and administrative controls can be demonstrated to be effective in limiting exposures to acceptable levels.

RECOMMENDATIONS
(CONTINUED)

1. Continue to use nitrile gloves for all the criminal investigation procedures.

2. Use chemical resistant clothing and safety glasses or goggles when working with chemicals and powders that have the potential to contact the skin or eyes.

3. Monitor uncontrolled carbon black exposures at a crime scene to determine whether respiratory protection is needed. Our data indicate that respirators are not required under the OSHA Respiratory Protection Standard [29 CFR 1910.134] because the exposures we measured in the crime lab were below applicable OELs. When they are working and used properly, engineering controls such as super glue fuming chambers and chemical fume hoods should adequately control irritating chemical odors. However, we recommend additional monitoring of carbon black exposures during the application of fingerprint powders at a crime scene (where engineering controls are not available). If these monitoring results are consistently below the OELs for carbon black, then this is a further indication that respirators are not required during this activity.

4. Consider making N95 filtering facepiece respirators available if respirators are to be used voluntarily, particularly where engineering controls cannot easily be implemented, such as during fingerprint powder application in the District 1 garage or at a crime scene. Although a written respiratory protection program is not mandatory for voluntary use, provide criminalists with a copy of Appendix D, "Information for Employees Using Respirators When Not Required Under the Standard," of the OSHA Respiratory Protection Standard [29 CFR 1910.134].

REFERENCES

ACGIH [2009]. Threshold limit values for chemical substances and physical agents and biological exposure indices. Cincinnati, OH: American Conference of Governmental Industrial Hygienists.

AIHA [2003]. ANSI/AIHA Standard Z9.5-2003, American National Standard for Laboratory Ventilation. Fairfax, VA: American Industrial Hygiene Association.

American Cancer Society [2009]. Cancer Facts & Figures 2009. [www.cancer.org/downloads/STT/500809web.pdf]. Date accessed: December 2009.

REFERENCES
(CONTINUED)

ASHRAE [2004]. ANSI/ASHRAE Standard 55-2004, Thermal Environmental Conditions for Human Occupancy. Atlanta, GA: American Society of Heating, Refrigerating and Air-Conditioning Engineers, Inc.

ASHRAE [2007a]. ANSI/ASHRAE Standard 62.1-2007, Ventilation for Acceptable Indoor Air Quality. Atlanta, GA: American Society of Heating, Refrigerating and Air-Conditioning Engineers, Inc.

ASHRAE [2007b]. Chapter 14, laboratories. In: 2007 ASHRAE handbook: heating, ventilating, and air-conditioning applications. Atlanta, GA: American Society of Heating, Refrigerating and Air-Conditioning Engineers, Inc.

Barni F, Lewis SW, Berti A, Miskelly GM, Lago G [2007]. Forensic application of the luminol reaction as a presumptive test for latent blood detection. Talanta 72(3):896–913.

CDC (Centers for Disease Control) [1990]. Guidelines for investigating clusters of health events. MMWR 39(11).

CFR. Code of Federal Regulations. Washington, DC: U.S. Government Printing Office, Office of the Federal Register.

FBI [2007]. Crime scene safety. In: Waggoner K, ed. Handbook of forensic services. Quantico, VA: U.S. Federal Bureau of Investigation, Laboratory Division, pp. 147–169.

Fingerprint Powder Accumulator [2005]. Model FPA TT-Tabletop. [http://home.att.net/~paytonscientific/page28.html]. Date accessed: December 2009.

Horswell J, ed. [2004]. The practice of crime scene investigation. Boca Raton, FL: CRC Press, p. 176.

IAI (International Association for Identification) [2004]. Safety Guidelines: Second Edition.

IPCS (WHO/International Programme on Chemical Safety) [1993]. International Chemical Safety Card: sodium bisulfite 38-40 aqueous solution. [www.cdc.gov/niosh/ipcsneng/neng1134.html]. Date accessed: December 2009.

REFERENCES
(CONTINUED)

Metz LM, McGuinness S [1997]. Responding to reported clusters of common diseases: the case of multiple sclerosis. Can J Public Health 88(4):277–279.

National Cancer Institute [2009] Surveillance Epidemiology and End Results. [http://seer.cancer.gov/statfacts/html/all.html]. Date accessed: December 2009.

NIOSH [1991]. Hazard evaluation and technical assistance report: Library of Congress, Washington. D.C. By Fine L, Teichman K. Cincinnati, OH: U.S. Department of Health and Human Services, Centers for Disease Control, National Institute for Occupational Safety and Health, NIOSH HETA Report No. 88-0364-2104.

NIOSH [1999]. Hazard evaluation and technical assistance report: State of Iowa Division of Narcotics Enforcement, Des Moines, Iowa. By Burton, NC. Cincinnati, OH: U.S. Department of Health and Human Services, Centers for Disease Control, National Institute for Occupational Safety and Health, NIOSH HETA Report No. 99-0252-2831.

Rugo HS [2004]. Occupational cancer. Chapter 16. In: La Dou J, ed. Current occupational and environmental medicine. 3rd rev. ed. New York: McGraw Hill Companies, Inc., pp. 229–267.

Carbon Dioxide, Temperature, and Relative Humidity Measurements

Carbon dioxide, temperature, and RH were monitored over time with a Q-Trak™ Plus (TSI Incorporated, Shoreview, Minnesota) direct reading monitor. These monitors were placed in the center of the occupied areas on the fourth, fifth, and sixth floors and set to collect data every 5 minutes.

Ventilation Measurements

TSI AccuBalance® flow hoods were used to measure the airflow through supply air diffusers and return air intakes. The TSI VelociCalc® Plus anemometer was used to measure air velocity through the LEV systems. Air velocity measurements were collected at approximately 4-inch intervals along the face of the LEV system or another opening where air was being drawn (e.g., open baffles on the super glue fuming chambers). The capture efficiency of the LEV systems was evaluated using irritant smoke tubes (Gastec Corporation, Kanagawa, Japan). To visualize the capture efficiency, smoke was generated in the work area where contaminants were to be captured or contained. Smoke tubes were also used to determine pressure differences by generating smoke near the doors of the rooms being evaluated and observing whether the smoke was drawn into the room (negative pressure) or pushed out of the room (positive pressure).

Air Sampling for Ethyl Acetate, Ammonia, Sulfur Dioxide, Carbon Black, and Hydrogen Peroxide

Pocket pumps (SKC Incorporated, Eighty Four, Pennsylvania) were used for drawing airflows of 1.5 and 2 liters per minute through sampling media, while SKC Aircheck 2000 pumps were used for drawing airflows of 200 cc/min through sampling media. All pumps were precalibrated and postcalibrated with the sampling media connected. Ethyl acetate was sampled using charcoal tubes (100 milligram/50 milligram) at a flow rate of 200 cc/min and analyzed using NIOSH Method 1457 [NIOSH 2009]. Ethyl cyanoacrylate was sampled using phosphoric acid treated XAD-7 tubes at a flow rate of 200 cc/min and analyzed using OSHA Method 55 [OSHA 1985]. Ammonia was sampled using sulfuric acid treated silica gel tubes at a flow rate of 200 cc/min and analyzed using a modified NIOSH Method 6016 [NIOSH 2009] where ion selective electrode analysis was used instead of ion conductivity detection chromatography. Sulfur dioxide was sampled using a 37-millimeter cartridge containing a sodium carbonate-treated cellulose filter and a 0.8 micrometer cellulose ester membrane prefilter at a flow rate of 1.5 liters per minute and analyzed using NIOSH Method 6004 [NIOSH 2009]. Carbon black was sampled using preweighed 37-millimeter diameter PVC filters at a flow rate of 2 liters per minute and analyzed using NIOSH Method 5000 [NIOSH 2009]. Sampling for hydrogen peroxide was conducted using colorimetric indicator tubes (Drager, Lubeck, Germany) and a handheld Drager Accuro pump.

Bulk Sampling

A bulk sample of the black fingerprint powder (Hi-Fi Volcano Latent Print Powder, Silk Black, BPP0916, Sirchie®, Youngsville, North Carolina) was collected in a 20-milliliter glass vial. The bulk sample was analyzed for PAHs by desorbing a 0.2 gram aliquot of the sample in carbon disulfide, sonicating for 30 minutes, and analyzing by full-scan gas chromatography/mass spectrometry.

References

NIOSH [2009]. NIOSH manual of analytical methods (NMAM®). 4th ed. Schlecht PC, O'Connor PF, eds. Cincinnati, OH: U.S. Department of Health and Human Services, Centers for Disease Control and Prevention, National Institute for Occupational Safety and Health, DHHS (NIOSH) Publication 94–113 (August, 1994); 1st Supplement Publication 96135, 2nd Supplement Publication 98–119; 3rd Supplement 2003–154. [www.cdc.gov/niosh/nmam/].

OSHA [1985]. OSHA method 55: methyl-2-cyanoacrylate and ethyl-2-cyanoacrylate. In: Sampling and analytical methods. Salt Lake City, Utah: U.S. Department of Labor, Occupational Safety and Health Administration, Organic Methods Evaluation Branch. [www.osha.gov/dts/sltc/methods/index.html].

In evaluating the hazards posed by workplace exposures, NIOSH investigators use both mandatory (legally enforceable) and recommended OELs for chemical, physical, and biological agents as a guide for making recommendations. OELs have been developed by Federal agencies and safety and health organizations to prevent the occurrence of adverse health effects from workplace exposures. Generally, OELs suggest levels of exposure to which most employees may be exposed up to 10 hours per day, 40 hours per week for a working lifetime without experiencing adverse health effects. However, not all employees will be protected from adverse health effects even if their exposures are maintained below these levels. A small percentage may experience adverse health effects because of individual susceptibility, a pre-existing medical condition, and/or a hypersensitivity (allergy). In addition, some hazardous substances may act in combination with other workplace exposures, the general environment, or with medications or personal habits of the employee to produce health effects even if the occupational exposures are controlled at the level set by the exposure limit. Also, some substances can be absorbed by direct contact with the skin and mucous membranes in addition to being inhaled, which contributes to the individual's overall exposure.

Most OELs are expressed as a TWA exposure. A TWA refers to the average exposure during a normal 8- to 10-hour workday. Some chemical substances and physical agents have recommended STEL or ceiling values where health effects are caused by exposures over a short period. Unless otherwise noted, the STEL is a 15-minute TWA exposure that should not be exceeded at any time during a workday, and the ceiling limit is an exposure that should not be exceeded at any time.

In the United States, OELs have been established by Federal agencies, professional organizations, state and local governments, and other entities. Some OELs are legally enforceable limits, while others are recommendations. The U.S. Department of Labor OSHA PELs (29 CFR 1910 [general industry]; 29 CFR 1926 [construction industry]; and 29 CFR 1917 [maritime industry]) are legal limits enforceable in workplaces covered under the Occupational Safety and Health Act. NIOSH RELs are recommendations based on a critical review of the scientific and technical information available on a given hazard and the adequacy of methods to identify and control the hazard. NIOSH RELs can be found in the *NIOSH Pocket Guide to Chemical Hazards* [NIOSH 2005]. NIOSH also recommends different types of risk management practices (e.g., engineering controls, safe work practices, employee education/training, personal protective equipment, and exposure and medical monitoring) to minimize the risk of exposure and adverse health effects from these hazards. Other OELs that are commonly used and cited in the U.S. include the TLVs recommended by ACGIH, a professional organization, and the WEELs recommended by the American Industrial Hygiene Association, another professional organization. The TLVs and WEELs are developed by committee members of these associations from a review of the published, peer-reviewed literature. They are not consensus standards. ACGIH TLVs are considered voluntary exposure guidelines for use by industrial hygienists and others trained in this discipline "to assist in the control of health hazards" [ACGIH 2009]. WEELs have been established for some chemicals "when no other legal or authoritative limits exist" [AIHA 2008].

Outside the United States, OELs have been established by various agencies and organizations and include both legal and recommended limits. Since 2006, the Berufsgenossenschaftliches Institut für Arbeitsschutz (German Institute for Occupational Safety and Health) has maintained a database of international OELs from European Union member states, Canada (Québec), Japan, Switzerland, and the United States available at www.dguv.de/bgia/en/gestis/limit_values/index.jsp. The database contains international limits for over 1250 hazardous substances and is updated annually.

Employers should understand that not all hazardous chemicals have specific OSHA PELs, and for some agents the legally enforceable and recommended limits may not reflect current health-based information. However, an employer is still required by OSHA to protect its employees from hazards even in the absence of a specific OSHA PEL. OSHA requires an employer to furnish employees a place of employment free from recognized hazards that cause or are likely to cause death or serious physical harm [Occupational Safety and Health Act of 1970 (Public Law 91–596, sec. 5(a)(1))]. Thus, NIOSH investigators encourage employers to make use of other OELs when making risk assessment and risk management decisions to best protect the health of their employees. NIOSH investigators also encourage the use of the traditional hierarchy of controls approach to eliminate or minimize identified workplace hazards. This includes, in order of preference, the use of: (1) substitution or elimination of the hazardous agent, (2) engineering controls (e.g , local exhaust ventilation, process enclosure, dilution ventilation), (3) administrative controls (e.g., limiting time of exposure, employee training, work practice changes, medical surveillance), and (4) personal protective equipment (e.g., respiratory protection, gloves, eye protection, hearing protection). Control banding, a qualitative risk assessment and risk management tool, is a complementary approach to protecting employee health that focuses resources on exposure controls by describing how a risk needs to be managed. Information on control banding is available at www.cdc.gov/niosh/topics/ctrlbanding/. This approach can be applied in situations where OELs have not been established or can be used to supplement the OELs, when available.

Table 1 (on page 8) provides the OELs for each of the chemicals we monitored during this evaluation. Below, we discuss the potential health effects from exposure to the chemicals used for the different criminal investigation procedures. Although we could not sample every chemical used at the CPD, we sampled chemicals with greatest potential for exposure and/or the greatest potential to cause adverse health effects.

Black Fingerprint Powder Application

The black fingerprint powder used at the CPD (Hi-Fi Volcano Latent Print Powder, Silk Black, BPP0916, Sirchie, Youngsville, North Carolina) contains an unspecified amount of carbon black and lycopodium. Health hazard information was neither provided nor found in the literature for lycopodium. Carbon black is listed by IARC as a possible human carcinogen based on sufficient evidence in experimental animals, but inadequate evidence in humans [IARC 2006]. ACGIH lists carbon black as "not classifiable as a human carcinogen" [ACGIH 2001]. The ACGIH TLV applies only to commercially produced carbon black (not soot produced by combustion that may contain PAHs) and is intended to minimize complaints of dirtiness and accumulation of nontoxic dust in the pulmonary system [ACGIH 2001]. The NIOSH REL is reduced from 3.5 to 0.1 mg/m^3 if the carbon black contains PAHs [NIOSH 2005]. The reason for this lower limit is that PAHs are considered "carcinogenic to humans" [IARC 2008]. The carbon black used in the fingerprint powder at the CPD is commercial grade and does not contain PAHs. Thus, the reduced NIOSH REL does not apply.

Ninhydrin Spraying

The ninhydrin solution used at the CPD was a mixture of 10% acetone, 90% ethyl acetate, and dissolved ninhydrin crystals (triketohydrindene hydrate) supplied by Sirchie. Little information exists in the literature on potential health effects from ninhydrin exposure. Cases of allergic rhinitis and occupational asthma following dermal exposure to ninhydrin solution have been documented [Hytonen et al. 1996; Piirila et al. 1997]. Ninhydrin was sprayed inside a chemical fume hood. Because ninhydrin has a low vapor pressure (solid at room temperature) and the droplets formed during spraying settled quickly onto surfaces, the potential for dermal exposure may be greater than for inhalation exposure. For this reason, and due to a lack of air sampling methods, we did not collect PBZ air samples for ninhydrin. We did, however, observe glove use.

Acetone has higher OELs (e.g., ACGIH TLV = 500 ppm) than ethyl acetate (e.g., ACGIH TLV = 400 ppm), and the proportion of ethyl acetate was much greater than acetone in the ninhydrin solution. Therefore, we focused our air sampling efforts on ethyl acetate. The OELs for ethyl acetate are based primarily upon the potential irritating effects to the eyes, nose, skin, and upper airways [ACGIH 2001; NIOSH 2005].

Super Glue Fuming

Super glue is the common name for ethyl cyanoacrylate, which has an unpleasant, acrid odor. Neither OSHA nor NIOSH has issued OELs for ethyl cyanoacrylate. The ACGIH TLV is based upon the potential for eye, skin, and upper respiratory tract irritation, dermatitis, and possible respiratory sensitization or asthma [ACGIH 2001]. Although the TLV does not have a skin notation, skin contact has been shown to cause adhesions resulting in tissue damage [ACGIH 2001].

Luminol Spraying

Luminol solution used at the CPD (supplied by Sirchie) is an aqueous solution of sodium carbonate, sodium perborate tetrahydrate, and luminol (5-amino-2,3-dihydro-1,4-phthalazine-dione). Sodium carbonate is a base and sodium perborate tetrahydrate produces hydrogen peroxide in water. Health hazard information was neither provided nor found in the literature for luminol. Depending on the alkalinity of the luminol solution, skin irritation or chemical burns are possible. The OELs for hydrogen peroxide are based primarily on the potential irritating effects to the eyes, skin, mucous membranes, and respiratory tract [ACGIH 2001; NIOSH 2005]. In addition, ACGIH lists hydrogen peroxide as a "confirmed animal carcinogen with unknown relevance to humans" [ACGIH 2001].

Photo Processing

Several chemicals are used to develop and print photographs. Although many of the chemicals are contained in cartridges, some are poured into vats in the photo processing machine. Thus, the potential for dermal exposure to chemicals exists if protective clothing or gloves are not worn. In our review of the material safety data sheets, we found that ammonia (and ammonium containing compounds) and sodium bisulfite were present in the chemical formulations. Under heat, sodium bisulfite can decompose into sulfur dioxide [IPCS 1993]. The OELs for ammonia are based primarily on the potential for acute ocular damage and upper respiratory irritation, while the OELs for sulfur dioxide are based primarily on the potential for respiratory irritation and reductions in pulmonary function over time [ACGIH 2001; NIOSH 2005]. In addition, ammonia and sulfur dioxide have STELs of 5 and 35 ppm, respectively [NIOSH 2005; ACGIH 2009].

References

ACGIH [2001]. Documentation of the threshold limit values and biological exposure indices. 7th ed. Vol. I. Cincinnati, OH: American Conference of Governmental Industrial Hygienists.

ACGIH [2009]. Threshold limit values for chemical substances and physical agents and biological exposure indices. Cincinnati, OH: American Conference of Governmental Industrial Hygienists.

AIHA [2008]. AIHA 2008 Emergency response planning guidelines (ERPG) & workplace environmental exposure levels (WEEL) handbook. Fairfax, VA: American Industrial Hygiene Association.

CFR. Code of Federal Regulations. Washington, DC: U.S. Government Printing Office, Office of the Federal Register.

Hytonen M, Martimo KP, Estlander T, Tupasela O [1996]. Occupational IgE-mediated rhinitis caused by ninhydrin. Allergy 51(2):114–116.

IARC [2006]. IARC monographs on the evaluation of the carcinogenic risk to humans: carbon black. Lyon, France: World Health Organization, International Agency for Research on Cancer.

IARC [2008]. IARC monographs on the evaluation of the carcinogenic risk to humans: polycyclic aromatic hydrocarbons. Lyon, France: World Health Organization, International Agency for Research on Cancer.

IPCS (WHO/International Programme on Chemical Safety) [1993]. International Chemical Safety Card: sodium bisulfite 38-40 aqueous solution [www.cdc.gov/niosh/ipcsneng/neng1134.html]. Date accessed: April 2009.

NIOSH [2005]. NIOSH pocket guide to chemical hazards. Barsen ME, ed. Cincinnati, OH: U.S. Department of Health and Human Services, Centers for Disease Control and Prevention, National Institute for Occupational Safety and Health, DHHS (NIOSH) Publication No. 2005-149. [www.cdc.gov/niosh/npg/]. Date accessed: July 2009.

Piirila P, Estlander T, Hytonen M, Keskinen H, Tupasela O, Tuppurainen M [1997]. Rhinitis caused by ninhydrin develops into occupational asthma. Eur Respir J 10(8):1918–1921.

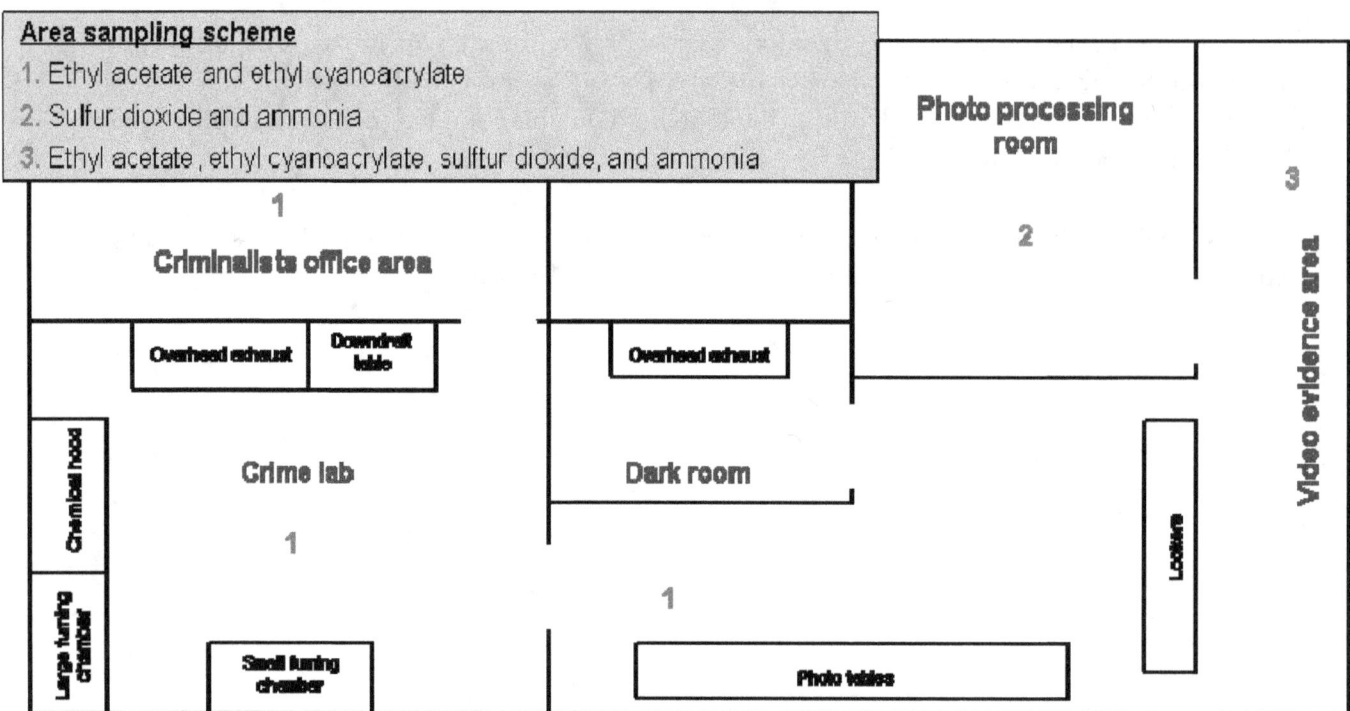

Figure C1. Area sampling locations and chemicals monitored at each location.

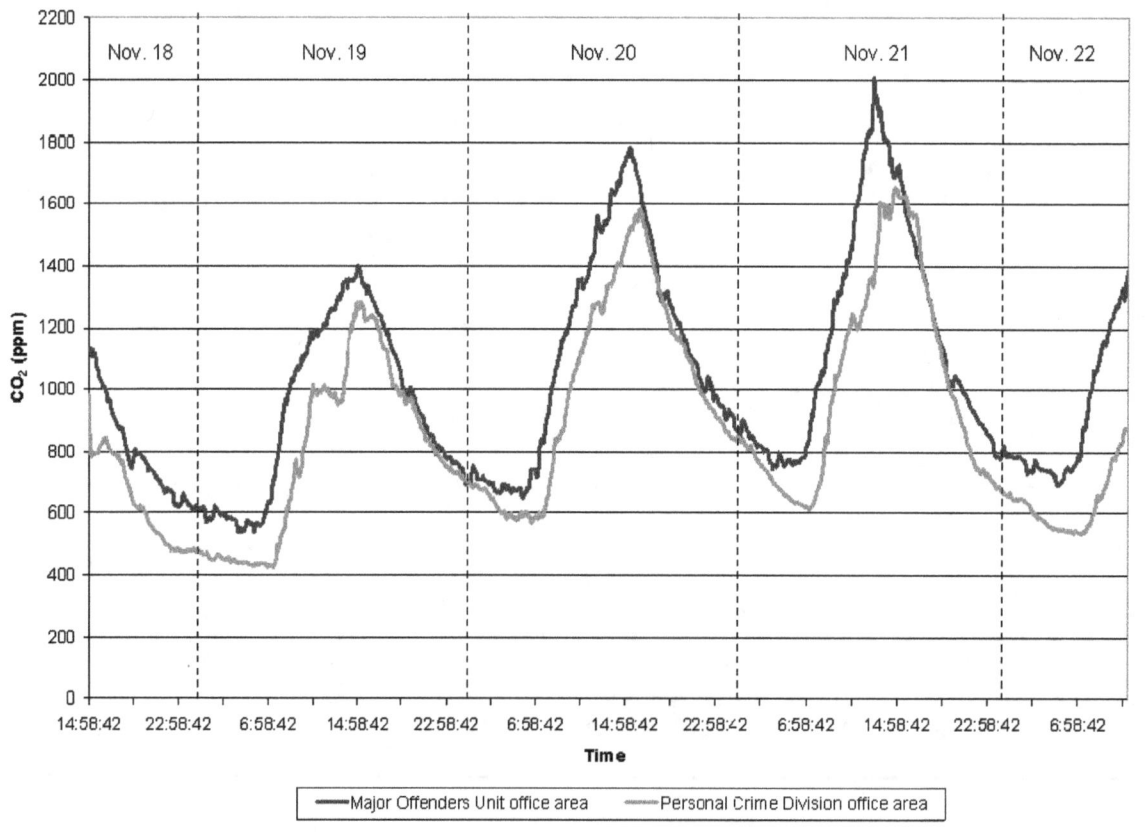

Figure C2. Carbon dioxide levels over time in the occupied office areas of the fourth floor.

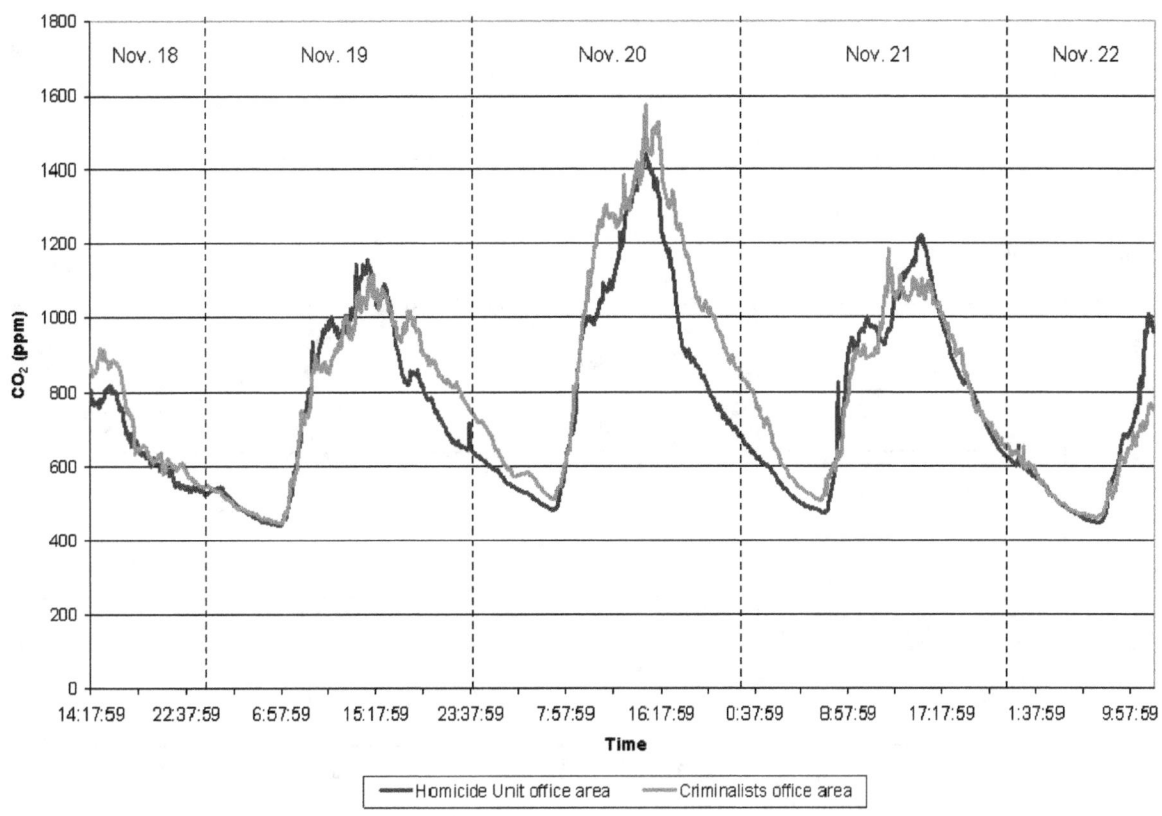

Figure C3. Carbon dioxide levels over time in the occupied office areas of the fifth floor.

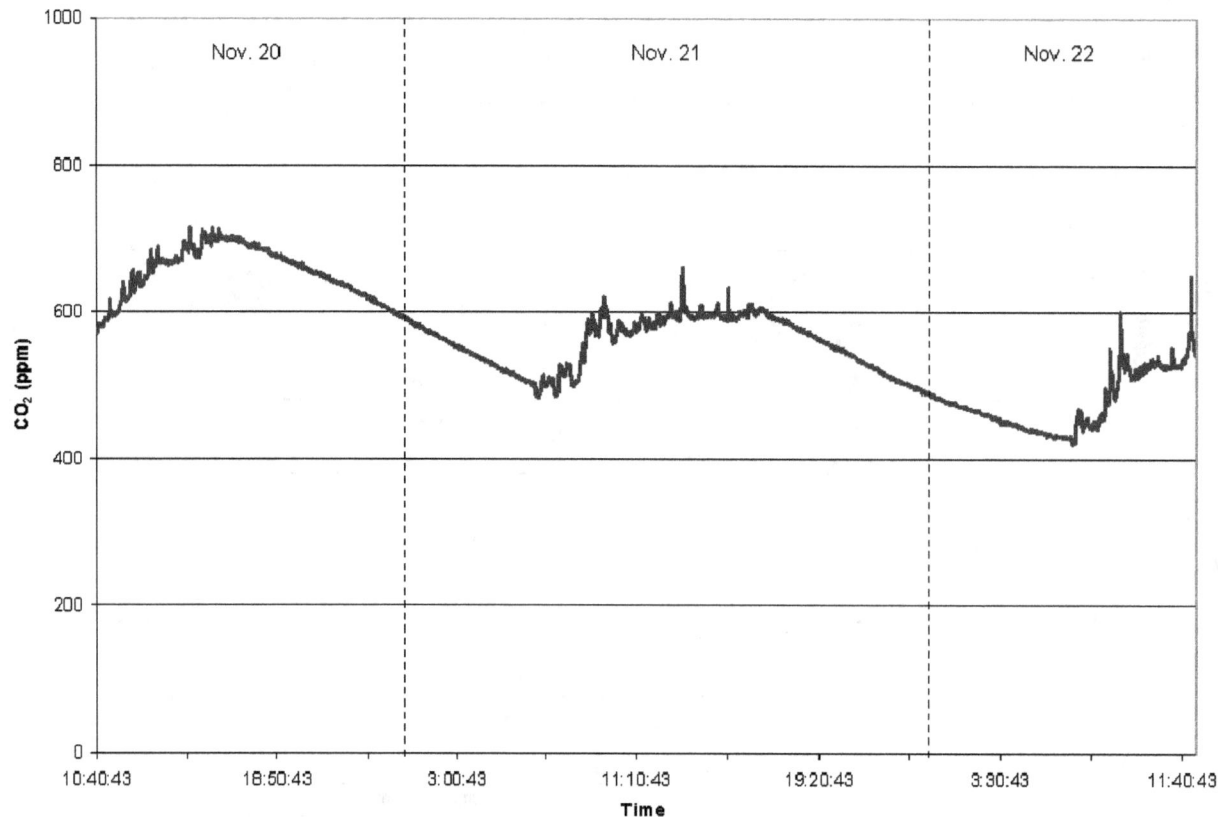

Figure C4. Carbon dioxide levels over time in the evidence room on the sixth floor.

ACKNOWLEDGMENTS AND AVAILABILITY OF REPORT

The Hazard Evaluations and Technical Assistance Branch (HETAB) of the National Institute for Occupational Safety and Health (NIOSH) conducts field investigations of possible health hazards in the workplace. These investigations are conducted under the authority of Section 20(a)(6) of the Occupational Safety and Health (OSHA) Act of 1970, 29 U.S.C. 669(a)(6) which authorizes the Secretary of Health and Human Services, following a written request from any employer or authorized representative of employees, to determine whether any substance normally found in the place of employment has potentially toxic effects in such concentrations as used or found. HETAB also provides, upon request, technical and consultative assistance to federal, state, and local agencies; labor; industry; and other groups or individuals to control occupational health hazards and to prevent related trauma and disease.

The findings and conclusions in this report are those of the authors and do not necessarily represent the views of NIOSH. Mention of any company or product does not constitute endorsement by NIOSH. In addition, citations to websites external to NIOSH do no constitute NIOSH endorsement of the sponsoring organizations or their programs or products. Furthermore, NIOSH is not responsible for the content of these websites. All Web addresses referenced in this document were accessible as of the publication date.

This report was prepared by Kenneth W. Fent and Anthony Almazan of HETAB, Division of Surveillance, Hazard Evaluations and Field Studies (DSHEFS). Industrial hygiene field assistance was provided by Greg Burr, Todd Niemeier, Srinivas Durgam, and Seung Hee Jang. Medical field assistance was provided by Elena Page. Health communication assistance was provided by Stefanie Evans. Editorial assistance was provided by Ellen Galloway. Desktop publishing was performed by Robin Smith.

Copies of this report have been sent to employee and management representatives at CPD, CIS, the state health department, and the OSHA Regional Office. This report is not copyrighted and may be freely reproduced. The report may be viewed and printed at www.cdc.gov/niosh/hhe. Copies may be purchased from the National Technical Information Service (NTIS) at 5825 Port Royal Road, Springfield, Virginia 22161.

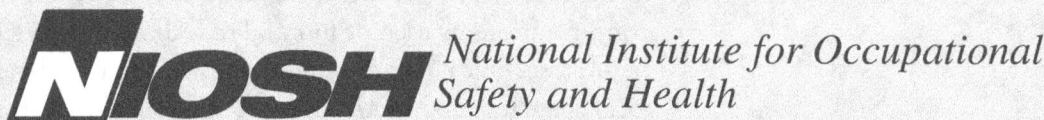
National Institute for Occupational Safety and Health

Delivering on the Nation's promise: Safety and health at work for all people through research and prevention.

To receive NIOSH documents or information about occupational safety and health topics, contact NIOSH at:

1-800-CDC-INFO (1-800-232-4636)

TTY: 1-888-232-6348

E-mail: cdcinfo@cdc.gov

or visit the NIOSH web site at: **www.cdc.gov/niosh**.

For a monthly update on news at NIOSH, subscribe to NIOSH eNews by visiting **www.cdc.gov/niosh/eNews**.

SAFER • HEALTHIER • PEOPLE™